The New Based Co of Fastest Recipes

How to Cook basically Anything from Easy Plant-Based Dishes

Levi Tonge

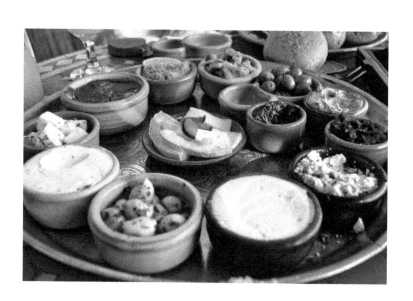

© **Copyright 2021- All rights reserved.**

The content contained within this book may not be reproduced, duplicated or transmitted without direct written permission from the author or the publisher. Under no circumstances will any blame or legal responsibility be held against the publisher, or author, for any damages, reparation, or monetary loss due to the information contained within this book. Either directly or indirectly.

Legal Notice:

This book is copyright protected. This book is only for personal use. You cannot amend, distribute, sell, use, quote or paraphrase any part, or the content within this book, without the consent of the author or publisher.

Disclaimer Notice:

Please note the information contained within this document is for educational and entertainment purposes only. All effort has been executed to present accurate, up to date, and reliable, complete information. No warranties of any kind are declared or implied. Readers acknowledge that the author is not engaging in the rendering of legal, financial, medical or professional advice. The content within this book has been derived from various sources. Please consult a licensed professional before attempting any techniques outlined in this book.

By reading this document, the reader agrees that under no circumstances is the author responsible for any losses, direct or indirect, which are incurred as a result of the use of information contained within this document, including, but not limited to, — errors, omissions, or inaccuracies.

Table of Contents

Hummus Without Oil

Servings: 6

Cooking Time: 0 Minutes

Ingredients:

- 2 tablespoons of lemon juice
- 1 15-ounce can of chickpeas
- 2 tablespoons of tahini
- 1-2 freshly chopped/minced garlic cloves
- Red pepper hummus
- 2 tablespoons of almond milk pepper

Directions:

1. Rinse the chickpeas and put them in a high-speed blender with garlic. Blend them until they break into fine pieces.

2. Add the other ingredients and blend everything until you have a smooth paste. Add some water if you want a less thick consistency.

3. Your homemade hummus dip is ready to be served with eatables!

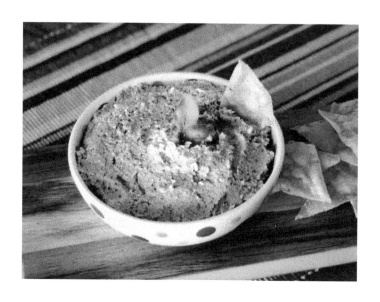

6

Kiwi & Peanut Bars

Servings: 9

Cooking Time: 5 Minutes **Ingredients:**

- 2 kiwis, mashed
- 1 tbsp maple syrup
- ½ tsp vanilla extract
- 2 cups old-fashioned rolled oats
- ½ tsp salt
- ¼ cup chopped peanuts

Directions:

1. Preheat oven to 360 F.

2. In a bowl, add kiwi, maple syrup, and vanilla and stir. Mix in oats, salt, and peanuts. Pour into a greased baking dish and bake for -30 minutes, until crisp. Let completely cool and slice into bars to serve.

Snickers Pie

Servings: 16

Cooking Time: 0 Minute

Ingredients:

- For the Crust:
- 12 Medjool dates, pitted
- 1 cup dried coconut, unsweetened
- 5 tablespoons cocoa powder
- 1/2 teaspoon sea salt
- 1 teaspoon vanilla extract, unsweetened
- 1 cup almonds
- For the Caramel Layer:
- 10 Medjool dates, pitted, soaked for 10 minutes in warm water, drained
- 2 teaspoons vanilla extract, unsweetened
- 3 teaspoons coconut oil
- 3 tablespoons almond butter, unsalted
- For the Peanut Butter Mousse:
- 3/4 cup peanut butter
- 2 tablespoons maple syrup
- 1/2 teaspoon vanilla extract, unsweetened

- 1/8 teaspoon sea salt

- 28 ounces coconut milk, chilled

Directions:

1. Prepare the crust, and for this, place all its ingredients in a food processor and pulse for 3 to 5 minutes until the thick paste comes together.

2. Take a baking pan, line it with parchment paper, place crust mixture in it and spread and press the mixture evenly in the bottom, and freeze until required.

3. Prepare the caramel layer, and for this, place all its ingredients in a food processor and pulse for 2 minutes until smooth.

4. Pour the caramel on top of the prepared crust, smooth the top and freeze for 30 minutes until set.

5. Prepare the mousse and for this, separate coconut milk and its solid, then add solid from coconut milk into a food processor, add remaining

ingredients and then pulse for 1 minute until smooth.

6.   Top prepared mousse over caramel layer, and then freeze for 3 hours until set.

7.   Serve straight away.

Nutrition Info: Calories: 456 Cal; Fat: 33 g: Carbs: 37g; Protein: 8.3 g; Fiber: 5 g

Peanut Tofu Wrap

Servings: 4

Cooking Time: 5 Minutes

Ingredients:

- ¼ c. cilantro, finely chopped
- 1 c. of the following:
- Asian pear
- English cucumber
- 1 ½ t. lime zest
- 1 tbsp. of the following:
- rice vinegar
- canola oil
- 5 tbsp. peanut sauce
- 14 oz. tofu, extra firm
- 8 cabbage leaves

Directions:

1. Prepare cabbage leaves by washing and drying. Be sure to remove any stems or ribs.

2. Place the tofu on a paper towel-lined plate and blot to remove the extra moisture.

3. Set a big nonstick skillet over medium-high heat and place the oil. Once the oil is warm, add the tofu and crumble it to cook, stirring often. Wait for approximately 5 minutes or until the tofu turns golden brown. Remove from the heat and set to the side.

4. Mix well using a spatula the liquid ingredients, except the oil, and add the lime zest.

5. Add the sauce to the skillet and combine.

6. Place the cabbage leaves on the plates and spoon the tofu mixture into the center, topping it with cilantro, cucumber, and pear.

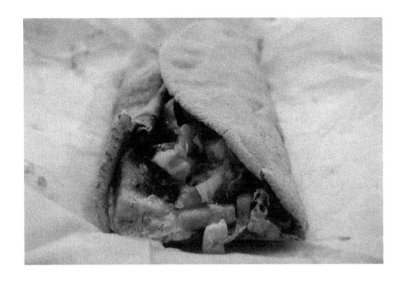

Coconut Cacao Bites

Servings: 20

Cooking Time: 0 Minute

Ingredients:

- 1 1/2 cups almond flour
- 3 dates, pitted
- 1 1/2 cups shredded coconut, unsweetened
- 1/4 teaspoons ground cinnamon
- 2 Tablespoons flaxseed meal
- 1/16 teaspoon sea salt
- 2 Tablespoons vanilla protein powder
- 1/4 cup cacao powder
- 3 Tablespoons hemp seeds
- 1/3 cup tahini
- 4 Tablespoons coconut butter, melted

Directions:

1. Place all the ingredients in a food processor and pulse for 5 minutes until the thick paste comes together.

2.   Drop the mixture in the form of balls on a baking sheet lined with parchment sheet, tablespoons per ball and then freeze for 1 hour until firm to touch.

3.   Serve straight away.

Nutrition Info: Calories: 120 Cal; Fat: 4.5 g: Carbs: 15 g; Protein: 4 g; Fiber: 2 g

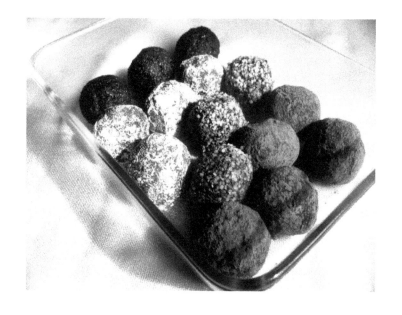

Roasted Apples Stuffed with Pecans & Dates

Servings: 4

Cooking Time: 40 Minutes

Ingredients:

- 4 apples, cored, halved lengthwise
- ½ cup finely chopped pecans
- 4 dates, pitted and chopped
- 1 tbsp plant butter
- 1 tbsp pure maple syrup
- ¼ tsp ground cinnamon

Directions:

1. Preheat oven to 360 F.

2. Mix the pecans, dates, butter, maple syrup, and cinnamon in a bowl. Arrange the apple on a greased baking pan and fill them with the pecan mixture. Pour 1 tbsp of water in the baking pan. Bake for 30-40 minutes, until soft and lightly browned. Serve immediately.

Keto Chocolate Brownies

Servings: 4

Cooking Time: 15 Minutes

Ingredients:

- ¼ t. of the following:
- salt
- baking soda
- ½ c. of the following:
- sweetener of your choice
- coconut flour
- vegetable oil
- water
- ¼ c. of the following:
- cocoa powder
- almond milk yogurt
- 1 tbsp. ground flax
- 1 t. vanilla extract

Directions:

1. Bring the oven to 350 heat setting.

2.   Mix the ground flax, vanilla, yogurt, oil, and water; set to the side for 10 minutes.

3.   Line an oven-safe 8x8 baking dish with parchment paper.

4.   After 10 minutes have passed, add coconut flour, cocoa powder, sweetener, baking soda, and salt.

5.   Bake for 1minutes; make sure that you placed it in the center. When they come out, they will look underdone.

6.   Place in the refrigerator and let them firm up overnight.

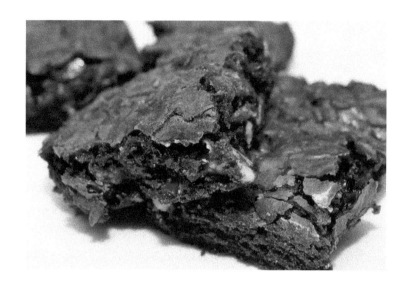

Raspberries & Cream Ice Cream

Servings: 4

Cooking Time: 0 Minutes

Ingredients:

- 2 Cups Raspberries
- 8 Oz. Coconut Cream
- 2 Tbsps. Coconut Flour
- 1 Tsp Maple Syrup
- 4-8 Raspberries for Filling

Directions:

1. Mix all ingredients in food processor and blend until well combined.

2. Spoon mixture into silicone mold and with raspberries and freeze for about 4 hours.

3. Remove balls from freezer and pop them out of the molds.

4. Serve immediately and enjoy!

Nutrition Info: Protein: 5% 12 kcal Fat: 69% 170 kcal

Carbohydrates: 26% 63 kcal

Vanilla Cinnamon Pudding

Servings: 4

Cooking Time: 25 Minutes

Ingredients:

- 1 cup basmati rice, rinsed
- 1 cup water
- 3 cups almond milk
- 12 dates, pitted
- 1 teaspoon vanilla paste
- 1 teaspoon ground cinnamon

Directions:

1. Add the rice, water and ½ cups of milk to a saucepan. Cover the saucepan and bring the mixture to a boil.

2. Turn the heat to low; let it simmer for another 10 minutes until all the liquid is absorbed.

3. Then, add in the remaining ingredients and stir to combine. Let it simmer for 10 minutes more or until the pudding has thickened. Bon appétit!

Nutrition Info: Per Serving: Calories: 332; Fat: 4.4g; Carbs: 64g; Protein: 9.9g

Mango & Papaya After-chop

Servings: 1

Cooking Time: 0 Minute

Ingredients:

- ¼ of papaya, chopped
- 1 mango, chopped
- 1 Tbsp coconut milk
- ½ tsp maple syrup
- 1 Tbsp peanuts, chopped

Directions:

1. Cut open the papaya. Scoop out the seeds, chop. 2.

Peel the mango. Slice the fruit from the pit, chop.

3. Put the fruit in a bowl. Add remaining ingredients.
Stir to coat.

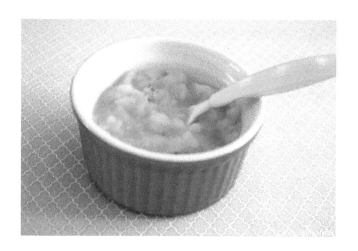

Curry Cauli Rice with Mushrooms

Servings: 4

Cooking Time: 15 Minutes

Ingredients:

- 8 oz baby bella mushrooms, stemmed and sliced
- 2 large heads cauliflower
- 2 tbsp toasted sesame oil, divided
- 1 onion, chopped
- 3 garlic cloves, minced
- Salt and black pepper to taste
- ½ tsp curry powder
- 1 tsp freshly chopped parsley
- 2 scallions, thinly sliced

Directions:

1.   Use a knife to cut the entire cauliflower head into 6 pieces and transfer to a food processor. With the grater
attachment, shred the cauliflower into a rice-like consistency.

2.   Heat half of the sesame oil in a large skillet over medium heat, and then add the onion and mushrooms. Sauté for 5 minutes or until the mushrooms are soft.

3.   Add the garlic and sauté for 2 minutes or until fragrant. Pour in the cauliflower and cook until the rice has slightly softened about 10 minutes.

4.   Season with salt, black pepper, and curry powder; then, mix the ingredients to be well combined. After, turn the heat off and stir in the parsley and scallions. Dish the cauli rice into serving plates and serve warm as a compliment for salads, barbecues, and soups.

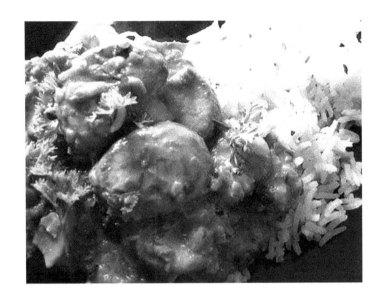

29

Cucumber Rounds with Hummus

Servings: 6

Cooking Time: 10 Minutes

Ingredients:

- 1 cup hummus, preferably homemade
- 2 large tomatoes, diced
- 1/2 teaspoon red pepper flakes
- Sea salt and ground black pepper, to taste
- 2 English cucumbers, sliced into rounds

Directions:

1. Divide the hummus dip between the cucumber rounds.

2. Top them with tomatoes; sprinkle red pepper flakes, salt and black pepper over each cucumber.

3. Serve well chilled and enjoy!

Nutrition Info: Per Serving: Calories: 88; Fat: 3.6g; Carbs: 11.3g; Protein: 2.6g

Servings: 4

Cooking Time: 20 Minutes

Ingredients:

- 3 oz dairy-free dark chocolate
- 1 tbsp coconut oil
- ½ cup pumpkin puree
- 2 tbsp pure date sugar
- ⅓ cup whole-wheat flour
- ½ tsp baking powder
- A pinch of salt

Directions:

1. Microwave chocolate and coconut oil for 90 seconds. Mix in pumpkin purée and sugar. Stir in flour, baking powder and salt. Pour the batter into ramekins. Arrange on a baking dish and pour in 2 cups of water. Bake for 20 minutes at 360 F. Let cool for a few minutes.
Serve topped with raspberries.

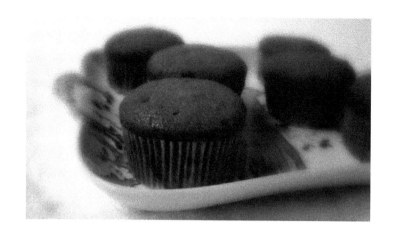

Double Chocolate Brownies

Servings: 9

Cooking Time: 25 Minutes

Ingredients:

- 1/2 cup vegan butter, melted
- 2 tablespoons applesauce
- 1/2 cup all-purpose flour
- 1/2 cup almond flour
- 1 teaspoon baking powder
- 2/3 cup brown sugar
- 1/2 teaspoon vanilla extract
- 1/3 cup cocoa powder
- A pinch of sea salt
- A pinch of freshly grated nutmeg
- 1/4 cup chocolate chips

Directions:

1. Start by preheating your oven to 350 degrees F.

2. In a mixing bowl, whisk the butter and applesauce until well combined. Then, stir in the remaining ingredients, whisking continuously to combine well.

3. Pour the batter into a lightly oiled baking pan. Bake in the preheated oven for about 25 minutes or until a tester inserted in the middle comes out clean.

4. Bon appétit!

Nutrition Info: Per Serving: Calories: 237; Fat: 14.4g;

Carbs: 26.5g; Protein: 2.8g

Caramel Brownie Slice

Servings: 16

Cooking Time: 0 Minute

Ingredients:

- For the Base:
- ¼ cup dried figs
- 1 cup dried dates
- ½ cup cacao powder
- ½ cup pecans
- ½ cup walnuts
- For the Caramel Layer:
- ¼ teaspoons sea salt
- 2 cups dried dates, soaked in water for 1 hour
- 3 Tablespoons coconut oil
- 5 Tablespoons water
- For the Chocolate Topping:
- 1/3 cup agave nectar
- ½ cup cacao powder
- ¼ cup of coconut oil

Directions:

1.   Prepare the base, and for this, place all its ingredients in a food processor and pulse for 3 to 5 minutes until the thick paste comes together.

2.   Take an 8 by 8 inches baking dish, grease it with oil, place base mixture in it and spread and press the mixture evenly in the bottom, and freeze until required.

3.   Prepare the caramel layer, and for this, place all its ingredients in a food processor and pulse for 2 minutes until smooth.

4.   Pour the caramel into the prepared baking dish, smooth the top and freeze for 20 minutes.

5.   Then prepare the topping and for this, place all its ingredients in a food processor, and pulse for 1 minute until combined.

6.   Gently spread the chocolate mixture over the caramel layer and then freeze for 3 hours until set.

7.   Serve straight away.

Nutrition Info: Calories: 128 Cal; Fat: 12 g: Carbs: 16 g; Protein: 2 g Fiber: 3 g

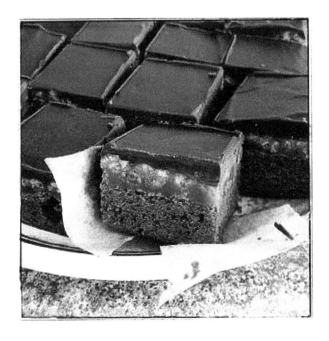

Nori Snack Rolls

Servings: 4

Cooking Time: 10 Minutes

Ingredients:

•   2 tablespoons almond, cashew, peanut, or others nut butter

•   2 tablespoons tamari, or soy sauce

•   4 standard nori sheets

•   1 mushroom, sliced

•   1 pickled ginger •   ½ cup grated carrots

Directions:

1.   Preparing the Ingredients.

2.   Preheat the oven to 350°F.

3.   Mix together the nut butter and tamari until smooth and very thick. Lay out a nori sheet, rough side up, the long way.

4.   Spread a thin line of the tamari mixture on the far end of the nori sheet, from side to side. Lay the mushroom slices, ginger, and carrots in a line at the other end (the end closest to you).

5. Fold the vegetables inside the nori, rolling toward the tahini mixture, which will seal the roll. Repeat to make 4 rolls.

6. Put on a baking sheet and bake for 8 to 10 minutes, or until the rolls are slightly browned and crispy at the ends. Let the rolls cool for a few minutes, then slice each roll into 3 smaller pieces.

Nutrition Info: Calories: 79; Total fat: 5g; Carbs: 6g; Fiber: 2g; Protein: 4g

Mango And Banana Shake

Servings: 2

Cooking Time: 0 Minutes

Ingredients:

- 1 Banana, Sliced and Frozen
- 1 Cup Frozen Mango Chunks
- 1 Cup Almond Milk
- 1 Tbsp. Maple Syrup
- 1 Tsp Lime Juice
- 2-4 Raspberries for Topping
- Mango Slice for Topping

Directions:

1. In blender, pulse banana, mango with milk, maple syrup, lime juice until smooth but still thick

2. Add more liquid if needed.

3. Pour shake into 2 bowls.

4. Top with berries and mango slice.

5. Enjoy!

Nutrition Info: Protein: 5% 8 kcal Fat: 11% 18 kcal
Carbohydrates: 85% 140 kcal

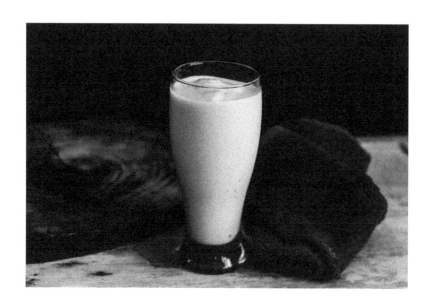

Coconut And Blueberries Ice Cream

Servings: 4

Cooking Time: 0 Minutes

Ingredients:

- 1/4 Cup Coconut Cream
- 1 Tbsp. Maple Syrup
- ¼ Cup Coconut Flour
- 1 Cup Blueberries
- ¼ Cup Blueberries for Topping

Directions:

1. Put ingredients into food processor and mix well on high speed.

2. Pour mixture in silicon molds and freeze in freezer for about 4 hours.

3. Once balls are set remove from freezer.

4. Top with berries.

5. Serve cold and enjoy!

Nutrition Info: Protein: 3% 4 kcal Fat: 40% 60 kcal

Carbohydrates: 57% 86 kcal

Apple and Pear Cobbler

Servings: 6

Cooking Time: 30 Minutes

Ingredients:

- Granny Smith apples, peeled, cored, and shredded
  - 2 ripe pears, peeled, cored, and cut into 1/4-inch slices
- 2 teaspoons fresh lemon juice
- ½ cup plus 2 tablespoons light brown sugar
- 2 tablespoons cornstarch
- 1 teaspoon ground cinnamon
- ½ teaspoon ground allspice
- 1 cup whole-grain flour
- 1½ teaspoons baking powder
- ¼ teaspoon salt
- 2 tablespoons canola or other neutral oil
- ½ cup plain or vanilla soy milk

Directions:

1. Preparing the Ingredients

2. Preheat the oven to 400°F. Grease a 9-inch square baking pan. Spread the apples and pears in the prepared pan. Sprinkle with the lemon juice and toss to coat. Stir in ½ cup of the sugar, cornstarch, cinnamon, and allspice while stirring to mix.

3. In a medium bowl, combine the flour, the remaining 2 tablespoons sugar, baking powder, and salt. Add the oil and mix with a fork until the mixture resembles coarse crumbs. Mix in the soy milk.

4. Bake

5. Spread the topping over the fruit. Bake until golden for about 30 minutes. Serve warm.

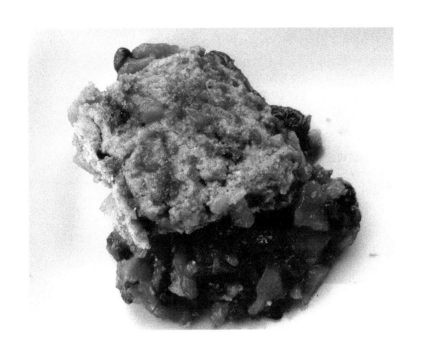

Chocolate Chip Banana Pancake

Servings: 6

Cooking Time: 10 Minutes

Ingredients:

- 1 large ripe banana, mashed
- 2 tablespoons coconut sugar
- 3 tablespoons coconut oil, melted
- 1 cup coconut milk
- 1 ½ cups whole wheat flour
- 1 teaspoon baking soda
- ½ cup vegan chocolate chips
- Olive oil, for frying

Directions:

1. Grab a large bowl and add the banana, sugar, oil and milk. Stir well.

2. Add the flour and baking soda and stir again until combined.

3. Add the chocolate chips and fold through then pop to one side.

4.   Place a skillet over a medium heat and add a drop of oil.

5.   Pour ¼ of the batter into the pan and move the pan to cover.

6.   Cook for 3 minutes then flip and cook on the other side.

7.   Repeat with the remaining pancakes then serve and enjoy.

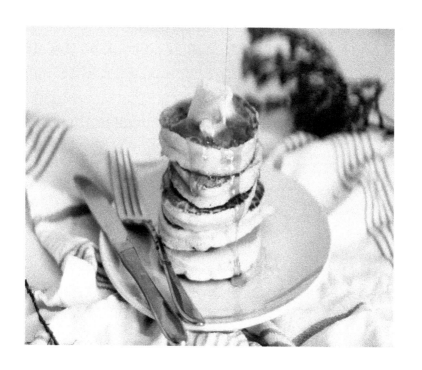

Strawberry Parfaits with Cashew Crème

Servings: 4

Cooking Time: 50 Minutes

Ingredients:

- ½ cup unsalted raw cashews
- 4 tablespoons light brown sugar
- ½ cup plain or vanilla soy milk
- ¾ cup firm silken tofu, drained
- 1 teaspoon pure vanilla extract
- 2 cups sliced strawberries
- 1 teaspoon fresh lemon juice
- Fresh mint leaves, for garnish

Directions:

1. Preparing the Ingredients

2. In a blender, grind the cashews and 3 tablespoons of the sugar to a fine powder. Add the soy milk and blend until smooth. Add the tofu and vanilla, then continue to

blend until smooth and creamy. Scrape the cashew mixture into a medium bowl, cover, and refrigerate for

30 minutes.

3. In a large bowl, combine the strawberries, lemon juice, and remaining 1 tablespoon sugar. Stir gently to combine and set aside at room temperature for 20 minutes.

4. Finish and Serve

5. Spoon alternating layers of the strawberries and cashew crème into parfait glasses or wineglasses, ending with a dollop of the cashew crème. Garnish with mint leaves and serve.

Donuts

Servings: 2

Cooking Time: 18 Minutes

Ingredients:

- 3 cups cherries, pitted, halved
- 1/2 teaspoon almond extract, unsweetened
- 2 tablespoons maple syrup
- 4 tablespoons granola
- 1 tablespoon almond butter melted

Directions:

1. Switch on the air fryer, insert the fryer basket, then shut it with the lid, set the frying temperature 350 degrees F, and let it preheat for 5 minutes.

2. Meanwhile, take a large ramekin, place cherries in it, and then stir in almond extract, butter and maple syrup until mixed.

3. Open the preheated fryer, place ramekin in it, close the lid and cook for 15 minutes until cooked, stirring halfway.

4.   When done, the air fryer will beep, open the lid, top cherries with granola, and then continue cooking for

3 minutes until the top has turned brown.

5.   Serve straight away.

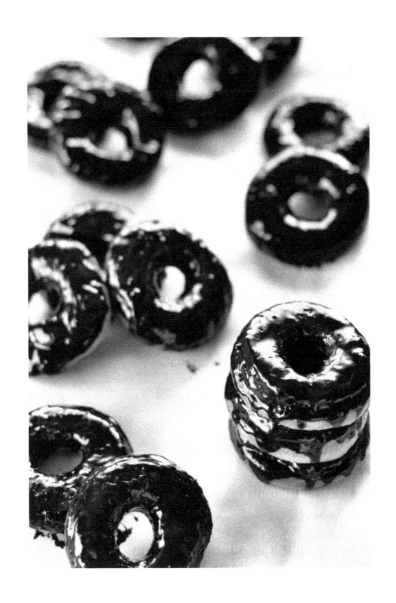

Parmesan Croutons with Rosemary Tomato Soup

Servings: 6

Cooking Time: 1 Hour 25 Minutes

Ingredients:

- 3 tbsp flax seed powder
- 1 ¼ cups almond flour
- 2 tsp baking powder
- 5 tbsp psyllium husk powder
- tsp plain vinegar
- 3 oz plant butter
- 2 grated plant-based Parmesan
- 2 lb fresh ripe tomatoes
- 4 cloves garlic, peeled only
- 1 small white onion, diced
- 1 small red bell pepper, diced
- 3 tbsp olive oil
- 1 cup coconut cream
- ½ tsp dried rosemary
- ½ tsp dried oregano
- 2 tbsp chopped fresh basil
- Salt and black pepper to taste

- Basil leaves to garnish

Directions:

1.   In a medium bowl, mix the flax seed powder with 9 tbsp of water and set aside to soak for 5 minutes. Preheat oven to 350 F and line a baking sheet with parchment paper.

2.   In another bowl, combine almond flour, baking powder, psyllium husk powder, and salt. When the flax egg is ready, mix in 1 ¼ cups boiling water and plain vinegar. Add in the flour mixture and whisk for 30 seconds. Form 8 flat pieces out of the dough. Place the flattened dough on the baking sheet while leaving enough room between each to allow rising. Bake for 40 minutes. Remove the croutons to cool and break them into halves. Mix the plant butter with plant-based Parmesan cheese and spread the mixture in the inner parts of the croutons. Increase the oven's temperature to 450 F and bake the croutons further for 5 minutes or until golden brown and crispier.

3.   In a baking pan, add tomatoes, garlic, onion, red bell pepper, and drizzle with olive oil. Roast in the oven

for 25 minutes and after broil for to 4 minutes until some of the tomatoes are slightly charred transfer to a blender and add coconut cream, rosemary, oregano, basil, salt, and black pepper. Puree until smooth and creamy. Pour the soup into serving bowls, drop some croutons on top, garnish with basil leaves, and serve.

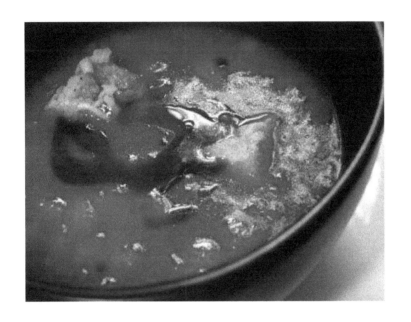

Lemon-maple Glazed Carrots

Servings: 4

Cooking Time: 15 Minutes

Ingredients:

- 1 lb baby carrots
- 2 tbsp plant butter
- 2 tbsp pure maple syrup
- 1 tbsp freshly squeezed lemon juice
- ½ tsp black pepper
- ¼ cup chopped fresh parsley

Directions:

1. Boil some water in a medium pot. Add some salt and cook the carrots until tender, 5 to 6 minutes. Drain the carrots. Melt the butter in a large skillet and mix in the maple syrup and lemon juice. Toss in the carrots, season with black pepper, and toss in the parsley. Serve the carrots.

Peanut Butter

Servings: 12

Cooking Time: 0 Minutes

Ingredients:

- 1½ cups vegan chocolate chips, divided
- ½ cup peanut butter, almond or cashew butter, or sunflower seed butter
- ¼ cup packed brown sugar
- 2 tablespoons nondairy milk

Directions:

1. Preparing the Ingredients.

2. Line the cups of a muffin tin with paper liners or reusable silicone cups.

3. In a small microwave-safe bowl, heat ¾ cup of the chocolate chips on high power for 1 minute. Stir. Continue heating in -second increments, stirring after each, until the chocolate is melted.

4. Pour about 1½ teaspoons of melted chocolate into each prepared muffin cup. Set aside, and allow them to harden.

5.   In a small bowl, stir together the peanut butter, brown sugar, and milk until smooth. Scoop about 1½ teaspoons of the mixture on top of the chocolate base in each cup. It's okay if the chocolate is not yet hardened.

6.   Finish and Serve

7.   Melt the remaining ¾ cup of chocolate chips using the directions in step 1. Pour another 1½ teaspoons of chocolate on top of the peanut butter in each cup, softly spreading it to cover. Let the cups sit until the chocolate hardens, about 15 minutes in the refrigerator or several hours on the counter. Leftovers will keep in the refrigerator for up to 2 weeks.

Nutrition Info: Per Serving: (1 cup) Calories 227; Protein: 4g; Total fat: 14g; Saturated fat: 6g; Carbohydrates: 22g; Fiber: 3g

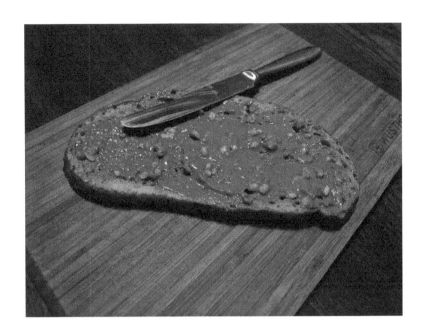

Almond Butter, Oat and Protein Energy Balls

Servings: 4

Cooking Time: 3 Minutes

Ingredients:

- 1 cup rolled oats
- ½ cup honey
- 2 ½ scoops of vanilla protein powder
- 1 cup almond butter
- Chia seeds for rolling

Directions:

1. Take a skillet pan, place it over medium heat, add butter and honey, stir and cook for 2 minutes until warm.

2. Transfer the mixture into a bowl, stir in protein powder until mixed, and then stir in oatmeal until combined.

3. Shape the mixture into balls, roll them into chia seeds, then arrange them on a cookie sheet and refrigerate for 1 hour until firm.

4.   Serve straight away

Nutrition Info: Calories: 200 Cal; Fat: 10 g: Carbs: 21 g; Protein: 7 fibers: 4 g

Stuffed Jalapeño Bites

Servings: 6

Cooking Time: 15 Minutes

Ingredients:

- 1/2 cup raw sunflower seeds, soaked overnight and drained
- 4 tablespoons scallions, chopped
- 1 teaspoon garlic, minced
- 3 tablespoons nutritional yeast
- 1/2 cup cream of onion soup
- 1/2 teaspoon cayenne pepper
- 1/2 teaspoon mustard seeds
- 12 jalapeños, halved and seeded
- 1/2 cup breadcrumbs

Directions:

1. In your food processor or high-speed blender, blitz raw sunflower seeds, scallions, garlic, nutritional yeast, soup, cayenne pepper and mustard seeds until well combined.

2.	Spoon the mixture into the jalapeños and top them with the breadcrumbs.

3.	Bake in the preheated oven at 400 degrees F for about 1minutes or until the peppers have softened. Serve warm.

4.	Bon appétit!

Nutrition Info: Per Serving: Calories: 108; Fat: 6.6g; Carbs: 7.3g; Protein: 5.3g

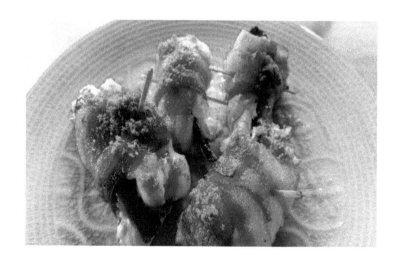

Easy Lebanese Toum

Servings: 6

Cooking Time: 10 Minutes

Ingredients:

- 2 heads garlic
- 1 teaspoon coarse sea salt
- 1 ½ cups olive oil
- 1 lemon, freshly squeezed
- 2 cups carrots, cut into matchsticks

Directions:

1. Puree the garlic cloves and salt in your food processor of a high-speed blender until creamy and smooth, scraping down the sides of the bowl.

2. Gradually and slowly, add in the olive oil and lemon juice, alternating between these two ingredients to create a fluffy sauce.

3. Blend until the sauce has thickened. Serve with carrot sticks and enjoy!

Nutrition Info: Per Serving: Calories: 252; Fat: 27g;

Carbs: 3.1g; Protein: 0.4g

Louisiana-style Sweet Potato Chips Servings: 4

Cooking Time: 55 Minutes

Ingredients:

- 2 sweet potatoes, peeled and sliced
- 2 tbsp melted plant butter
- 1 tbsp Cajun seasoning

Directions:

1. Preheat the oven to 400 F and line a baking sheet with parchment paper.

2. In a medium bowl, add the sweet potatoes, salt, plant butter, and Cajun seasoning. Toss well. Spread the chips on the baking sheet making sure not to overlap and bake in the oven for 50 minutes to 1 hour or until crispy. Remove the sheet and pour the chips into a large bowl.

Allow cooling and enjoy.

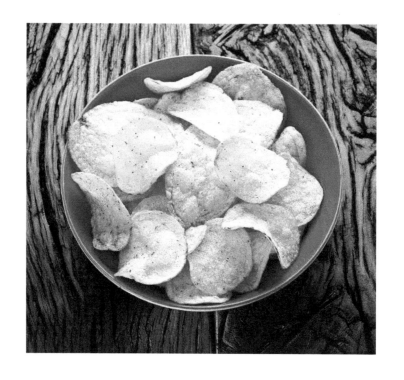

Peppery Hummus Dip

Servings: 10

Cooking Time: 10 Minutes

Ingredients:

- 20 ounces canned or boiled chickpeas, drained
- 1/4 cup tahini
- 2 garlic cloves, minced
- 2 tablespoons lemon juice, freshly squeezed
- 1/2 cup chickpea liquid
- 2 red roasted peppers, seeded and sliced
- 1/2 teaspoon paprika
- teaspoon dried basil
- Sea salt and ground black pepper, to taste
- 2 tablespoons olive oil

Directions:

1. Blitz all the ingredients, except for the oil, in your blender or food processor until your desired consistency is reached.

2. Place in your refrigerator until ready to serve.

3.   Serve with toasted pita wedges or chips, if desired.

Bon appétit!

Nutrition Info: Per Serving: Calories: 155; Fat: 7.9g; Carbs: 17.4g; Protein: 5.9g

Cherry Tomatoes with Hummus

Servings: 8

Cooking Time: 10 Minutes

Ingredients:

- 1/2 cup hummus, preferably homemade
- 2 tablespoons vegan mayonnaise
- 1/4 cup scallions, chopped
- 16 cherry tomatoes, scoop out pulp
- 2 tablespoons fresh cilantro, chopped
-

Directions:

1. In a mixing bowl, thoroughly combine the hummus, mayonnaise and scallions.

2. Divide the hummus mixture between the tomatoes. Garnish with fresh cilantro and serve.

3. Bon appétit!

Nutrition Info: Per Serving: Calories: 49; Fat: 2.5g; Carbs: 4.7g; Protein: 1.3g

Healthy Cauliflower Popcorn

Servings: 2

Cooking Time: 12 Hours

Ingredients:

- 2 heads of cauliflower
- Spicy Sauce
- ½ cup of filtered water
- ½ teaspoon of turmeric
- 1 cup of dates
- 2-3 tablespoons of nutritional yeast
- ¼ cup of sun-dried tomatoes
- 2 tablespoons of raw tahini
- 1-2 teaspoons of cayenne pepper
- 2 teaspoons of onion powder
- 1 tablespoon of apple cider vinegar
- 2 teaspoons of garlic powder

Directions:

1. Chop the cauliflower into small pieces so that you can have crunchy popcorn.

2. Put all the ingredients for the spicy sauce in a blender and create a mixture with a smooth consistency.

3. Coat the cauliflower florets in the sauce. See that each piece is properly covered.

4. Put the spicy florets in a dehydrator tray.

5. Add some salt and your favorite herb if you want.

6. Dehydrate the cauliflower for 12 hours at 115°F. Keep dehydrating until it is crunchy.

7. Enjoy the cauliflower popcorn, which is a healthier alternative!

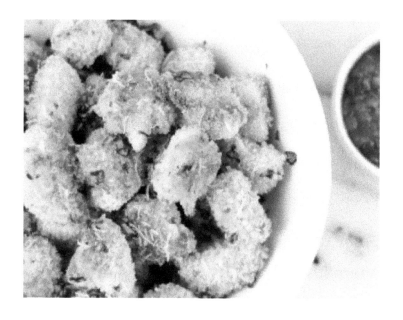

Maple Fruit Crumble

Servings: 4

Cooking Time: 25 Minutes

Ingredients:

*   3 cups chopped apricots
*   3 cups chopped mangoes
*   4 tbsp pure maple syrup
*   1 cup gluten-free rolled oats
*   ½ cup shredded coconut
*   2 tbsp coconut oil

Directions:

1. Preheat oven to 360 F.

2. Place the apricots, mangoes and tbsp of maple syrup in a round baking dish.

3. In a food processor, put the oats, coconut, coconut oil, and remaining maple syrup. Blend until combined. Pour over the fruit. Bake for 20-25 minutes. Allow to cool before slicing and serving.

Berry Compote with Red Wine

Servings: 4

Cooking Time: 15 Minutes

Ingredients:

*   4 cups mixed berries, fresh or frozen

*   1 cup sweet red wine

*   1 cup agave syrup

*   1/2 teaspoon star anise

*   1 cinnamon stick

*   3-4 cloves

*   A pinch of grated nutmeg

*   A pinch of sea salt

Directions:

1.   Add all ingredients to a saucepan. Cover with water by inch. Bring to a boil and immediately reduce the heat to a simmer.

2.   Let it simmer for 9 to 11 minutes. Allow it to cool completely.

3.   Bon appétit!

Nutrition Info: Per Serving: Calories: 260; Fat: 0.5g; Carbs: 64.1g; Protein: 1.1g

Avocado With Tahini Sauce

Servings: 4

Cooking Time: 10 Minutes

Ingredients:

- 2 large-sized avocados, pitted and halved
- 4 tablespoons tahini
- 4 tablespoons soy sauce
- 1 tablespoon lemon juice
- 1/2 teaspoon red pepper flakes
- Sea salt and ground black pepper, to taste
- 1 teaspoon garlic powder

Directions:

1. Place the avocado halves on a serving platter.

2. Mix the tahini, soy sauce, lemon juice, red pepper, salt, black pepper and garlic powder in a small bowl.

Divide the sauce between the avocado halves.

3. Bon appétit!

Nutrition Info: Per Serving: Calories: 304; Fat: 25.7g;

Carbs: 17.6g; Protein: 6g

Fruit And Almond Crisp

Servings: 8

Cooking Time: 45 Minutes

Ingredients:

- 4 cups peaches, pitted and sliced
- 3 cups plums, pitted and halved
- 1 tablespoon lemon juice, freshly squeezed
- 1 cup brown sugar
- For the topping:
- 2 cups rolled oats
- 1/2 cup oat flour
- 1 teaspoon baking powder
- 4 tablespoons water
- 1/2 cup almonds, slivered
- 1/2 teaspoon vanilla extract
- 1/2 teaspoon almond extract
- 1/4 teaspoon ground cloves
- 1/4 teaspoon ground cinnamon
- A pinch of kosher salt
- A pinch of grated nutmeg
- 5 ounces coconut oil, softened

Directions:

1.   Start by preheating your oven to 350 degrees F.

2.   Arrange the fruits on the bottom of a lightly oiled baking pan. Sprinkle lemon juice and 1/cup of brown sugar over them.

3.   In a mixing bowl, thoroughly combine the oats, oat flour, baking powder, water, almonds, vanilla, almond extract, ground cloves, cinnamon, salt, nutmeg and coconut oil.

4.   Spread the topping mixture over the fruit layer.

5.   Bake in the preheated oven for about 4minutes or until golden brown. Bon appétit!

Nutrition Info: Per Serving: Calories: 409; Fat: 19.1g;

Carbs: 55.6g; Protein: 7.7g

Chocolate And Avocado Pudding

Servings: 1

Cooking Time: 0 Minute

Ingredients:

- 1 small avocado, pitted, peeled
- 1 small banana, mashed
- 1/3 cup cocoa powder, unsweetened
- 1 tablespoon cacao nibs, unsweetened
- 1/4 cup maple syrup
- 1/3 cup coconut cream

Directions:

1. Add avocado in a food processor along with cream and then pulse for 2 minutes until smooth.

2. Add remaining ingredients, blend until mixed, and then tip the pudding in a container.

3. Cover the container with a plastic wrap; it should touch the pudding and refrigerate for hours.

4. Serve straight away.

Nutrition Info: Calories: 87 Cal; Fat: 7 g: Carbs: 9 g; Protein: 1.5 g; Fiber: 3.2 g

Easy Maple Rice Pudding

Servings: 4

Cooking Time: 30 Minutes

Ingredients:

*   1 cup short-grain brown rice

*   1 ¾ cups nondairy milk

*   4 tbsp pure maple syrup

*   1 tsp vanilla extract

*   A pinch of salt

*   ¼ cup dates, pitted and chopped

Directions:

1. In a pot over medium heat, place the rice, milk, ½ cups water, maple, vanilla, and salt. Bring to a boil, then reduce the heat. Cook for 20 minutes, stirring occasionally. Mix in dates and cook another 5 minutes. Serve chilled in cups.

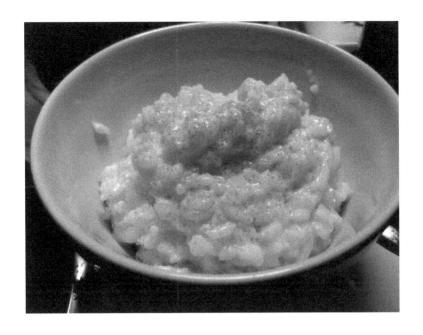

Coconut Yogurt Chia Pudding

Servings: 1

Cooking Time: 0 Minute

Ingredients:

- ½ cup vanilla coconut yogurt

- 2 tbsp chia seeds

- 3 tbsp almond milk

Directions:

1. Mix all ingredients in a bowl until well combined.

2. Place in the freezer for an hour or overnight.

3. When thickened, top with your favorite garnishes and serve.

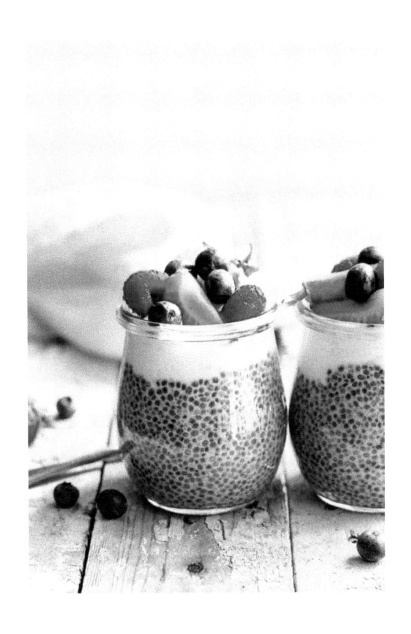

Orange Granita

Servings: 3

Cooking Time: 0 Minutes

Ingredients:

- ½cup light brown sugar
- ½cup water
- 2 cups orange juice
- 1 teaspoon fresh lemon juice

Directions:

1.   Preparing the Ingredients

2.   In a medium saucepan, combine the sugar and water and bring to a boil. Cook, stirring, until the sugar dissolves. Remove from heat and set aside to cool, about 15 minutes. Stir in the orange juice and lemon juice, then pour the mixture into a shallow baking pan.

3.   Cover and freeze until firm, stirring about once per hour, about hours.

4.   Finish and Serve

5.   When firm, remove the mixture from the freezer

and scrape it with the tines of a fork until fluffy. Spoon the granita into a container, cover, and freeze until serving time. The taste and texture of the granita is best if eaten within a few hours after it is made.

Brownie Energy Bites

Servings: 2

Cooking Time: 0 Minute

Ingredients:

- 1/2 cup walnuts
- 1 cup Medjool dates, chopped
- 1/2 cup almonds
- 18 teaspoon salt
- 1/2 cup shredded coconut flakes
- 1/3 cup and 2 teaspoons cocoa powder, unsweetened

Directions:

1. Place almonds and walnuts in a food processor and pulse for 3 minutes until the dough starts to come
together.

2. Add remaining ingredients, reserving ¼ cup of coconut and pulse for minutes until incorporated.

3.   Shape the mixture into balls, roll them in remaining coconut until coated, and refrigerate for 1 hour.

4.   Serve straight away

Nutrition Info: Calories: 174.6 Cal; Fat: 8.1 g: Carbs: 25.5 g; Protein: 4.1 g; Fiber: 4.4 g

Easy Mocha Fudge

Servings: 20

Cooking Time: 1 Hour 10 Minutes

Ingredients:

- 1 cup cookies, crushed
- 1/2 cup almond butter
- 1/4 cup agave nectar
- 6 ounces dark chocolate, broken into chunks
- 1 teaspoon instant coffee
- A pinch of grated nutmeg
- A pinch of salt

Directions:

1. Line a large baking sheet with parchment paper.

2. Melt the chocolate in your microwave and add in the remaining ingredients; stir to combine well.

3. Scrape the batter into a parchment-lined baking sheet. Place it in your freezer for at least 1 hour to set.

4. Cut into squares and serve. Bon appétit!

Nutrition Info: Per Serving: Calories: 105; Fat: 5.6g; Carbs: 12.9g; Protein: 1.1g

Strawberry Mousse

Servings: 4

Cooking Time: 15 Minutes

Ingredients:

- 8 ounces coconut milk, unsweetened
- 2 tablespoons honey
- 5 strawberries

Directions:

1. Place berries in a blender and pulse until the smooth mixture comes together.

2. Place milk in a bowl, whisk until whipped, and then add remaining ingredients and stir until combined.

3. Refrigerate the mousse for 10 minutes and then serve.

Nutrition Info: Calories: 145 Cal; Fat: 23 g: Carbs: 15 g; Protein: 5 g; Fiber: 1 g

Strawberries Stuffed whit Banana Cream

Servings: 4

Cooking Time: 10 Minutes

Ingredients:

- 12 strawberries, heads removed
- ¼ cup cashew cream
- ¼ tsp banana extract
- 1 tbsp unsweetened coconut flakes

Directions:

1.   Use a teaspoon to scoop out some of the strawberries pulp to create a hole within. In a small bowl, mix the cashew cream, banana extract, and maple syrup. Spoon the mixture into the strawberries and garnish with the coconut flakes. Serve.

Brownie Batter

Servings: 4

Cooking Time: 0 Minute

Ingredients:

- 4 Medjool dates, pitted, soaked in warm water
- 1.5 ounces chocolate, unsweetened, melted
- 2 tablespoons maple syrup
- 4 tablespoons tahini
- ½ teaspoon vanilla extract, unsweetened
- 1 tablespoon cocoa powder, unsweetened
- 1/8 teaspoon sea salt
- 1/8 teaspoon espresso powder
- 2 to 4 tablespoons almond milk, unsweetened

Directions:

1. Place all the ingredients in a food processor and process for 2 minutes until combined.

2. Set aside until required.

Nutrition Info: Calories: 44 Cal; Fat: 1g: Carbs: 6g; Protein: 2g Fiber: 0 g

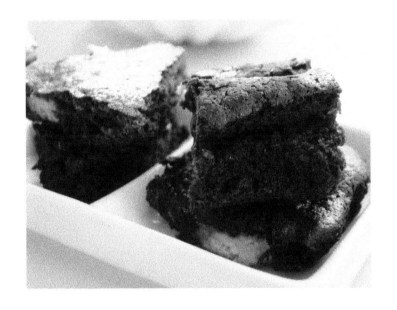

Chocolate Peppermint Mousse

Servings: 4

Cooking Time: 10 Minutes

Ingredients:

- ¼ cup Swerve sugar, divided
- 4 oz cashew cream cheese, softened
- 3 tbsp cocoa powder
- ¾ tsp peppermint extract
- ½ tsp vanilla extract
- 1/3 cup coconut cream

Directions:

1. Put 2 tablespoons of Swerve sugar, cashew cream cheese, and cocoa powder in a blender. Add the peppermint extract, ¼ cup warm water, and process until smooth. In a bowl, whip vanilla extract, coconut cream, and the remaining Swerve sugar using a whisk. Fetch out 5-6 tablespoons for garnishing. Fold in the cocoa mixture

until thoroughly combined. Spoon the mousse into serving cups and chill in the fridge for 30 minutes. Garnish with the reserved whipped cream and serve immediately.

Banana Mango Ice Cream

Servings: 2

Cooking Time: 0 Minute

Ingredients:

- 1 banana, peeled and sliced
- 2 ripe mangos with the skin removed and the flesh cubed
- 3 tablespoons almond or cashew milk, chilled

Directions:

1. Lay out the banana and mango slices on a baking sheet lined with parchment paper and place them in the freezer.

2. Once they are frozen solid, remove the fruit and place it in the food processor.

3. Add the cold milk and process until smooth, about three to four minutes.

4. Taste and add sweetener as needed.

5. Serve immediately.

Spiced Roasted Cauliflower
Servings: 6

Cooking Time: 25 Minutes

Ingredients:

*   1 ½ pounds cauliflower florets

*   1/4 cup olive oil

*   4 tablespoons apple cider vinegar

*   2 cloves garlic, pressed

*   1 teaspoon dried basil

*   1 teaspoon dried oregano

*   Sea salt and ground black pepper, to taste

1. Arrange the cauliflower florets on a parchment lined baking sheet. Bake the cauliflower florets in the preheated oven for about 25 minutes or until they are
slightly charred.

2. Begin by preheating your oven to 420 degrees F.

Directions:

3. Toss the cauliflower florets with the remaining ingredients.

4.   Bon appétit!

Nutrition Info: Per Serving: Calories: 115; Fat: 9.3g;
Carbs: 6.9g; Protein: 5.6g

Healthy Protein Bars

Servings: 12

Cooking Time: 0 Minutes

Ingredients:

- 1 large banana
- 1 cup of rolled oats
- 1 serving of vegan vanilla protein powder

Directions:

1. In a food processor, blend the protein powder and rolled oats.

2. Blend them for 1 minute until you have a semicoarse mixture. The oats should be slightly chopped, but not powdered.

3. Add the banana and form a pliable and coarse dough.

4. Shape into either balls or small bars and store them in a container.

5. Eat one and store the rest in an airtight container in the refrigerator!

Arugula & Hummus Pitas

Servings: 4

Cooking Time: 15 Minutes

Ingredients:

- 1 garlic clove, chopped
- ¾ cup tahini
- 2 tbsp fresh lemon juice
- Salt to taste
- ⅛ tsp ground cayenne
- ¼ cup water
- 1 (15.5-oz) can chickpeas
- 2 medium carrots, grated
- 4 pita breads, whole wheat, halved
- 1 large ripe tomato, sliced
- 2 cups arugula

Directions:

1. In a food processor, add in garlic, tahini, lemon juice, salt, cayenne pepper, and water. Pulse until smooth. In a bowl, mash the chickpeas with a fork. Stir in carrots

and tahini mixture; reserve. Spread the hummus over the pitas and top with a tomato slice and

arugula. Serve immediately.

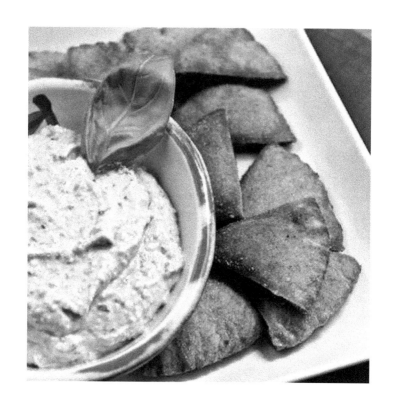

Lightning Source UK Ltd.
Milton Keynes UK
UKHW020802160621
385600UK00005B/68

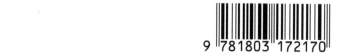